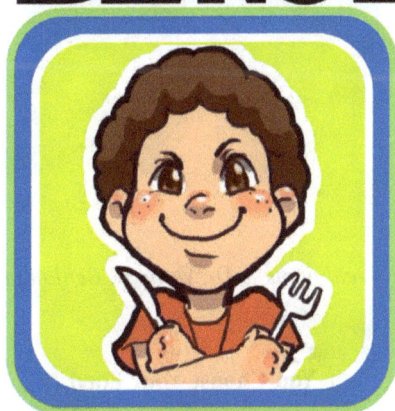

Healthy
BENJI

You Choose
Your Food

Dr. Benji's real name is Dr. Verna R. Benjamin-Lambert

You Choose Your Food

© 2012 by Dr. Verna R. Benjamin-Lambert

Library of Congress Control Number: 1817813

ISBN: 978-0-9910361-5-8

Printed in the United States of America

YOU CHOOSE YOUR FOOD

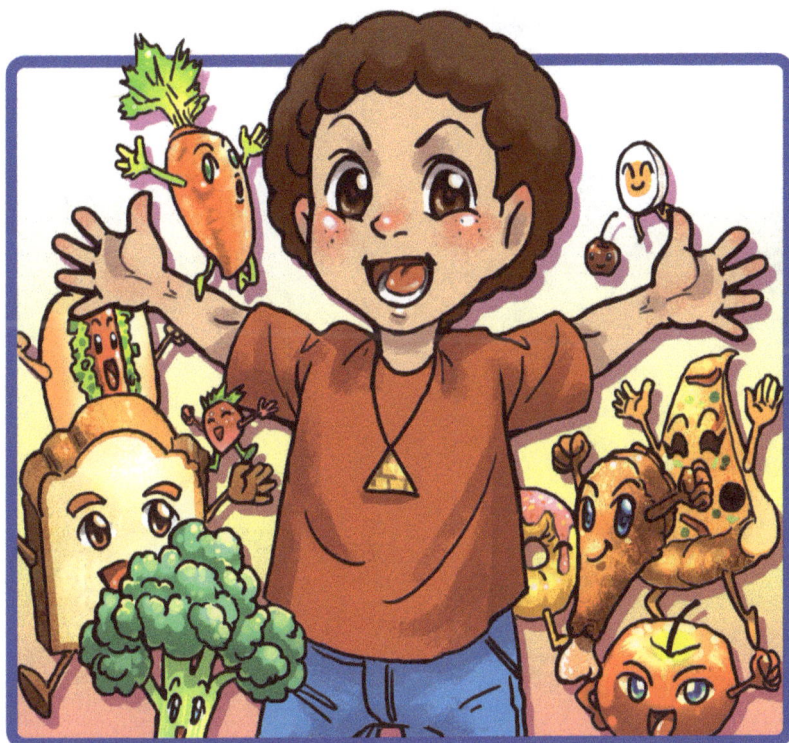

BY
DR. BENJI
ILLUSTRATED BY ARASHI YANG

HEALTHY READING FOR HEALTHY EATING!
BOOK FOR EARLY READERS

Health Intelligence, LLC.

To Parents and Teachers

The Healthy Benji book series brings excitement through reading about a variety of nutritious foods. Children will learn the value of various fruits and vegetables and understand how to make strategic choices as they nourish their bodies. The stories are designed to expose children to a wide array of food choices and for them to enjoy being a part of the preparation process.

Questions are asked at the end of each story to ensure that children understand and gain knowledge from what is read. Teachers and parents are encouraged to assist children in preparing meals using fresh fruits and vegetables to make dishes that children will find enjoyable to prepare and delicious to eat. When children become a part of the preparation process they will be more likely to try new things.

Throughout the Healthy Benji books series meaningful family connections are emphasized along with friendship, responsibility, manners, helpfulness, hygiene, appreciation and respect for others.

The Healthy Benji Book Series will help children develop healthy eating habits at a very early age. Through reading about and practicing healthy habits our children will have the best foundation possible to enjoy a wholesome and happy life.

LET'S START HERE! IT'S COOL TO BE HEALTHY

Healthy Benji was hungry.
He went to the kitchen.

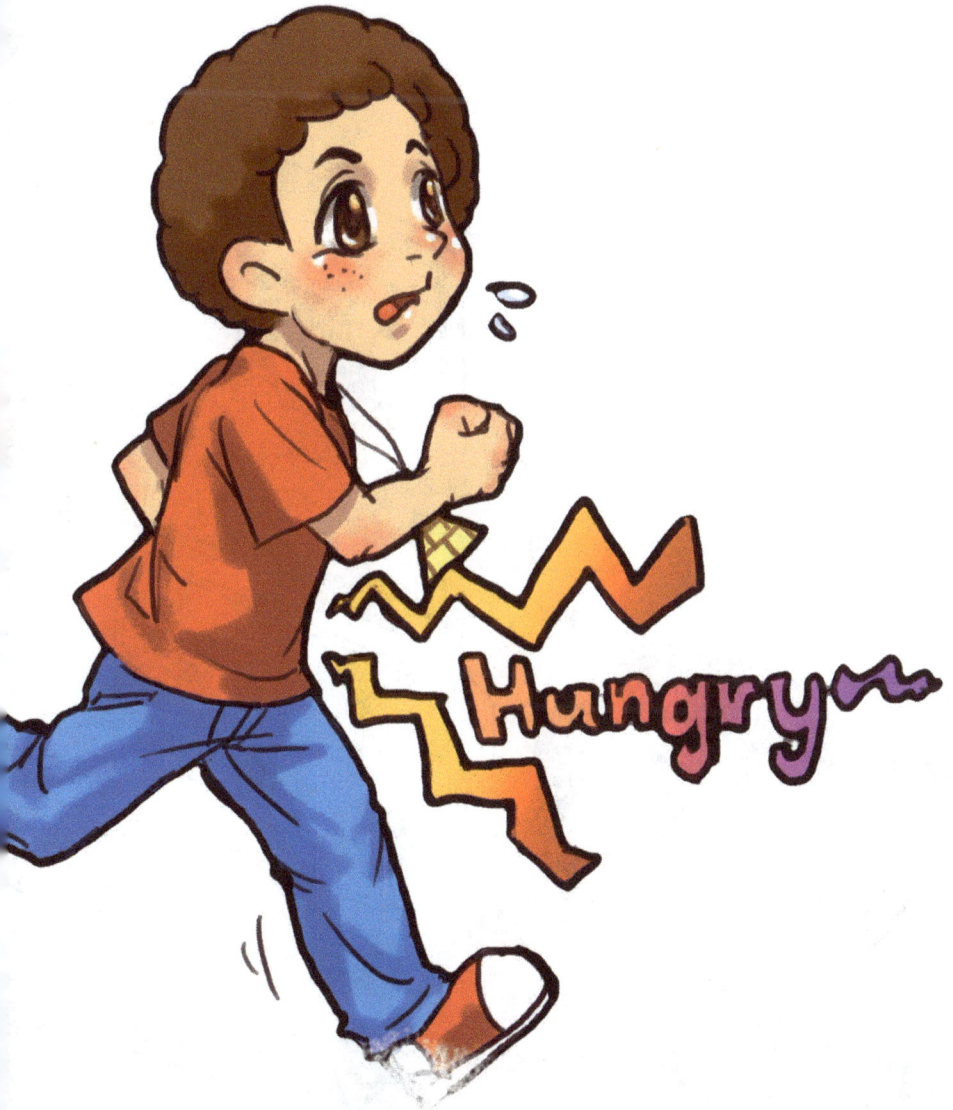

When he opened the
refrigerator, he heard a voice
that said, "Do you need a
treat?" It was a plump juicy
plum on the top shelf.

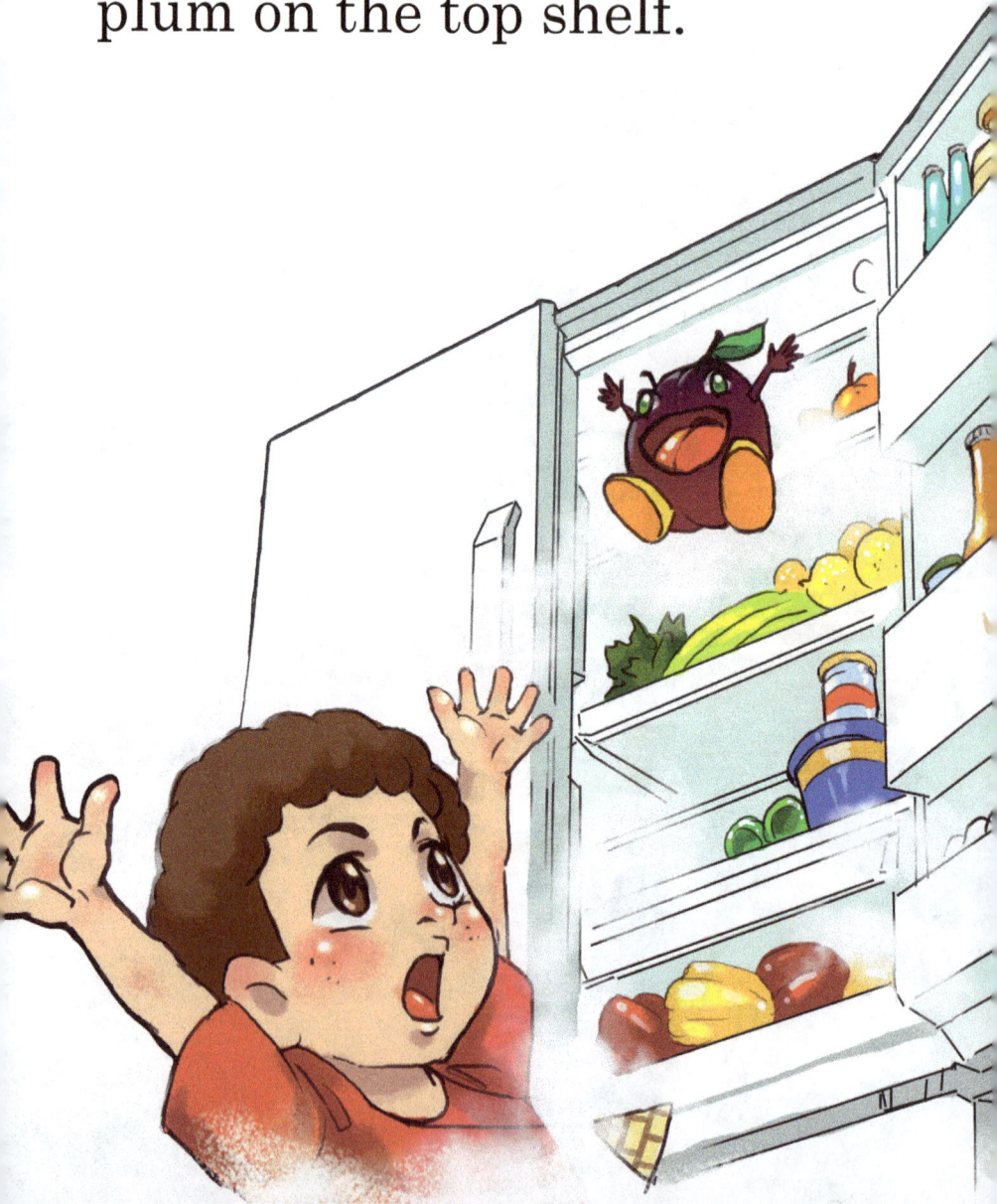

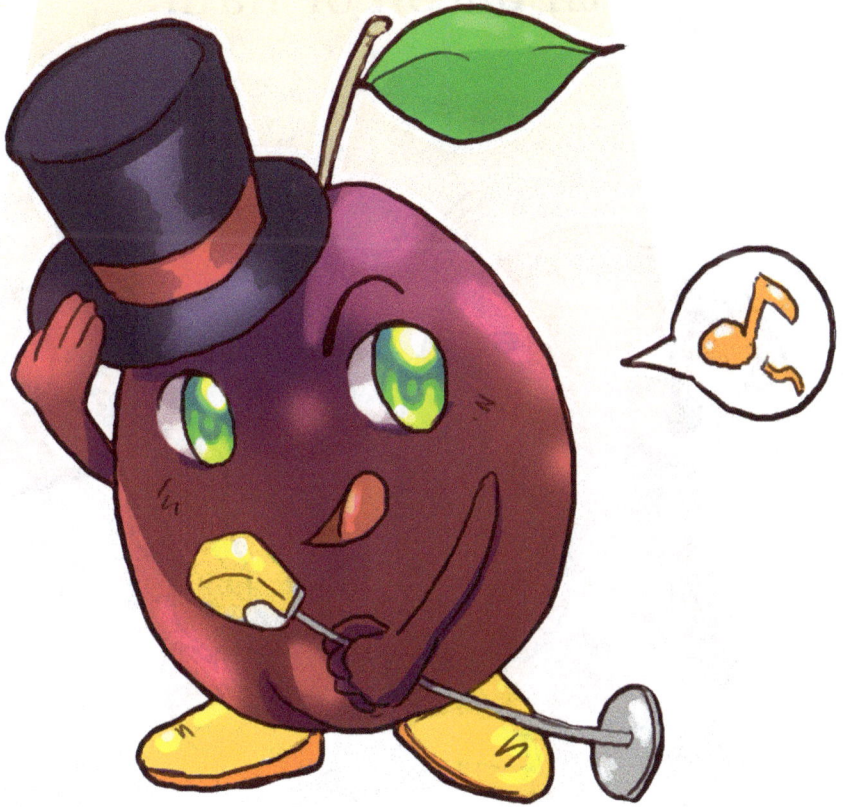

"Do you want to eat?
Do you want a treat?"

You can choose
sweet potato pancakes
with bacon or ham.

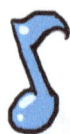

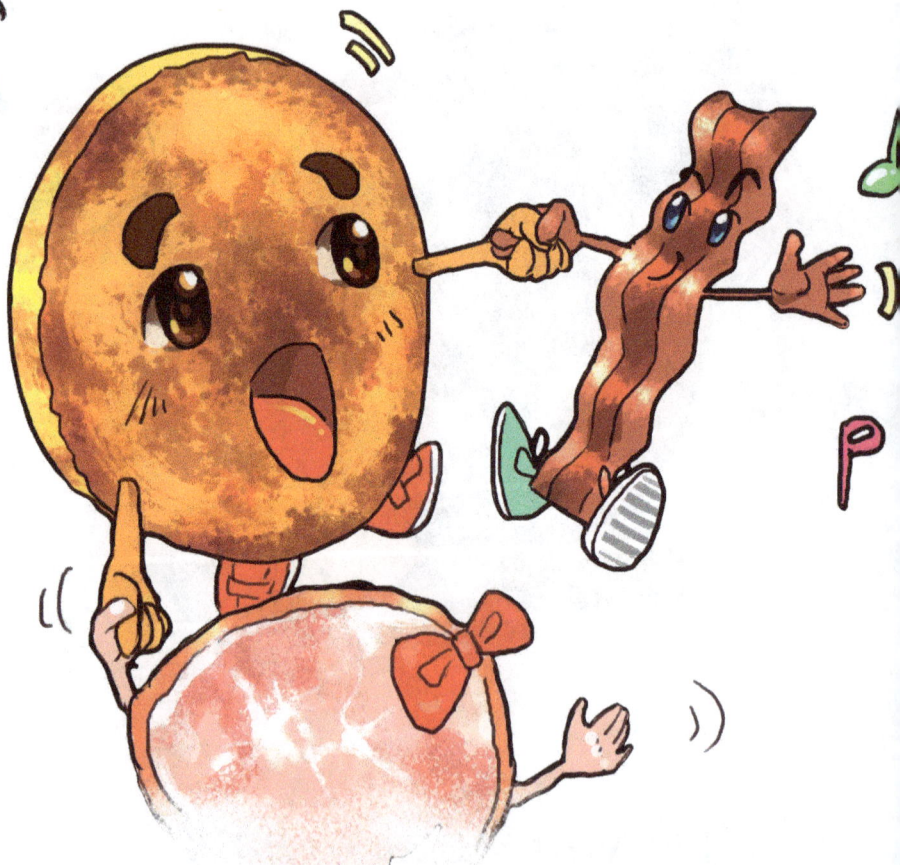

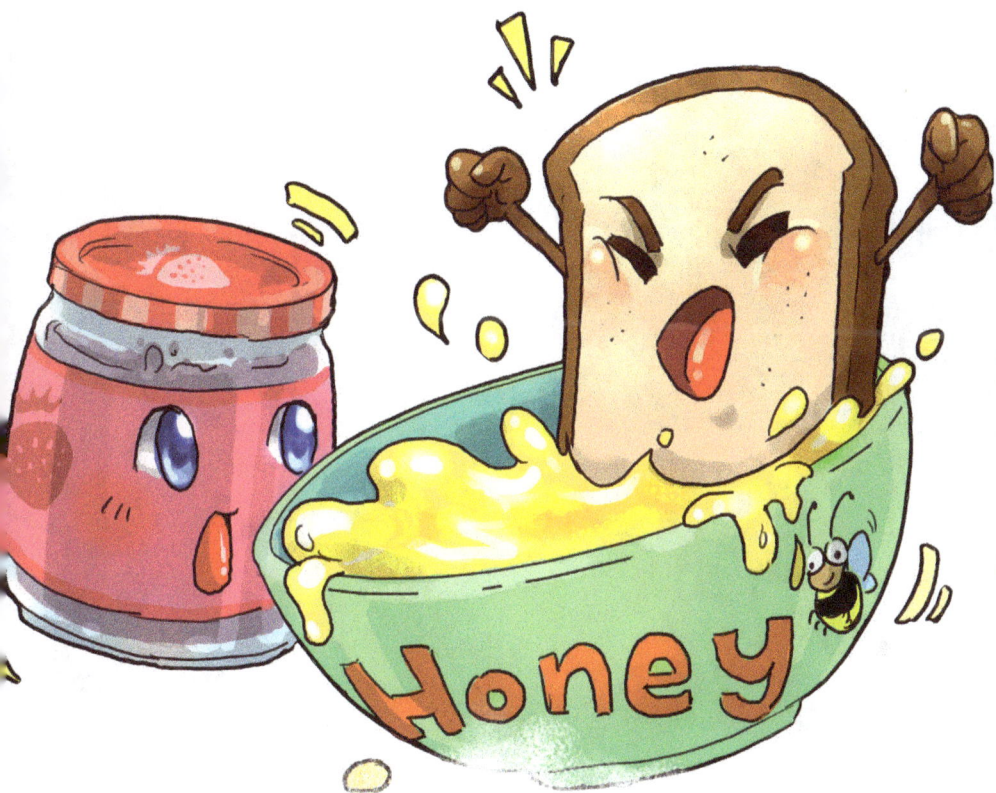

You can have
wheat toast with
honey or jam.

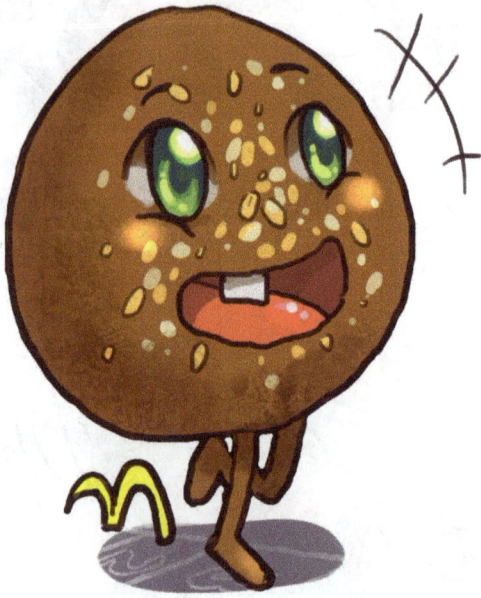

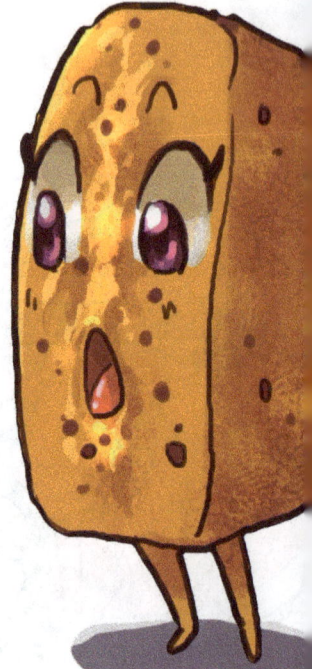

You can choose oatmeal
or banana bread.

You can choose blueberry muffins or bagels.

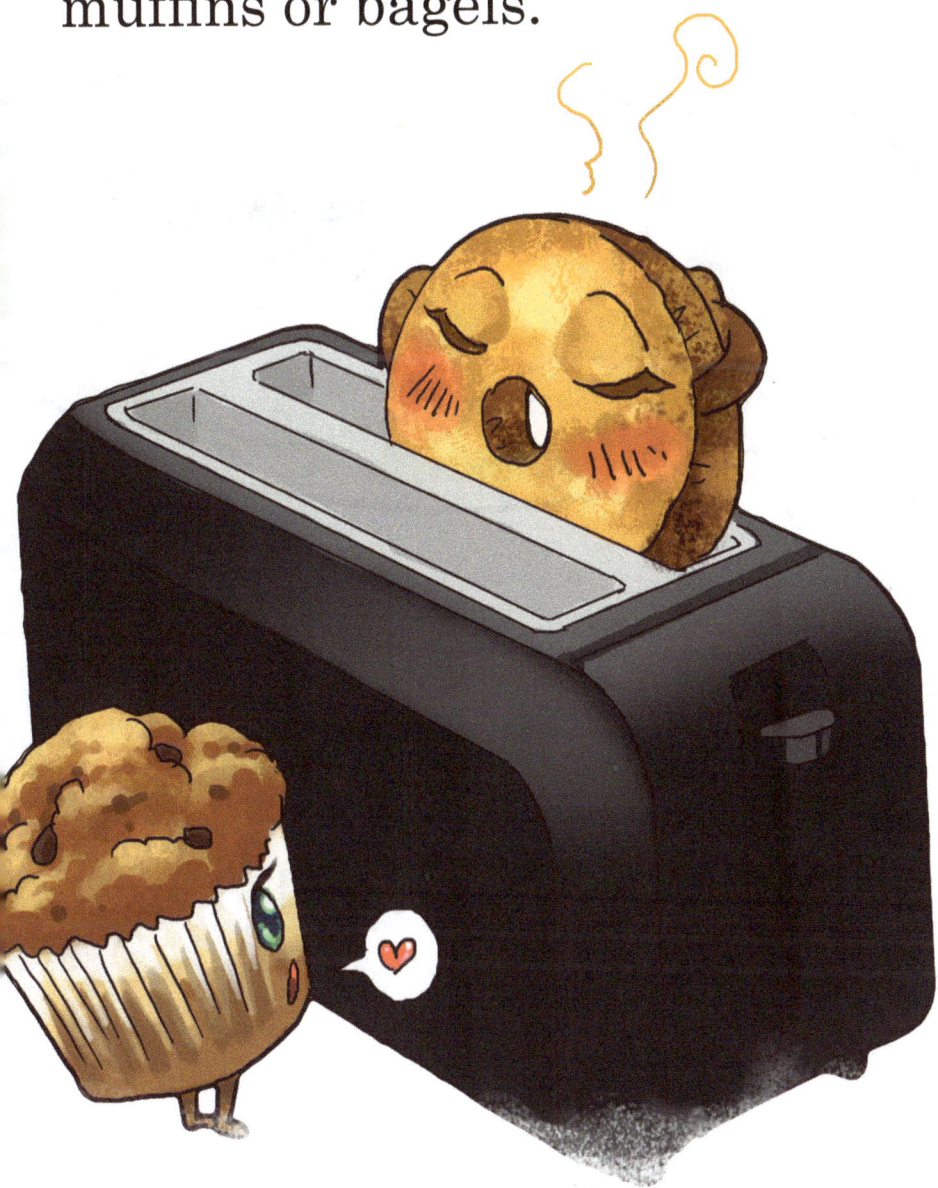

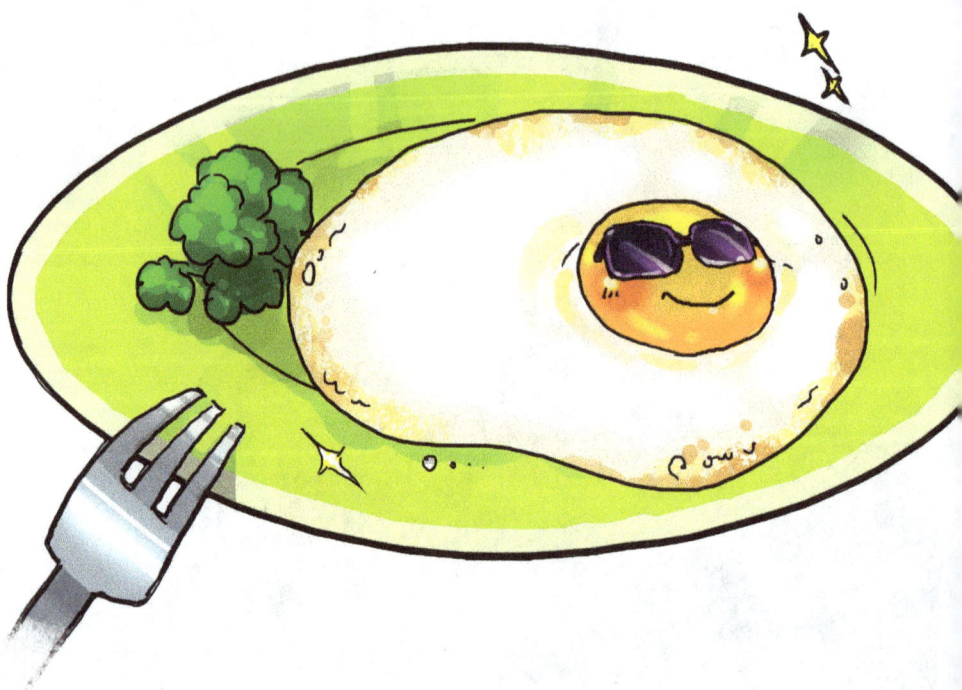

You can eat scrambled eggs, or yogurt.

You can choose crunchy
veggies, or fresh fruit

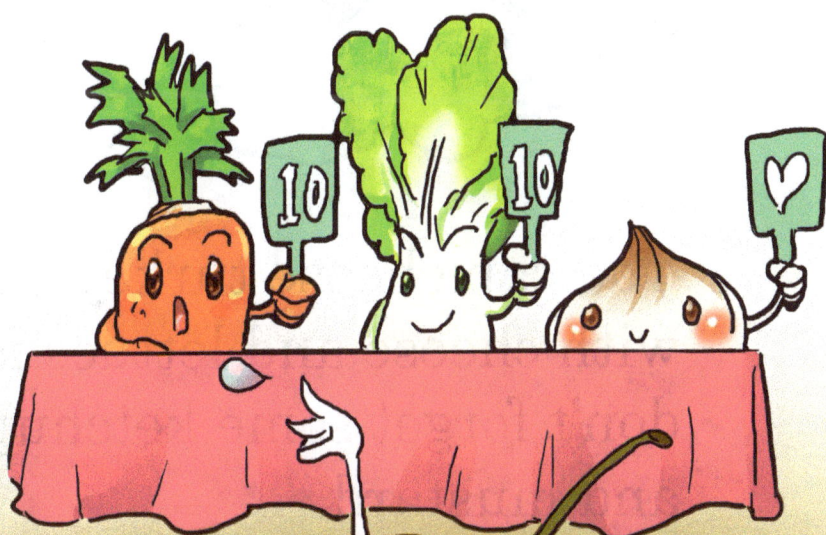

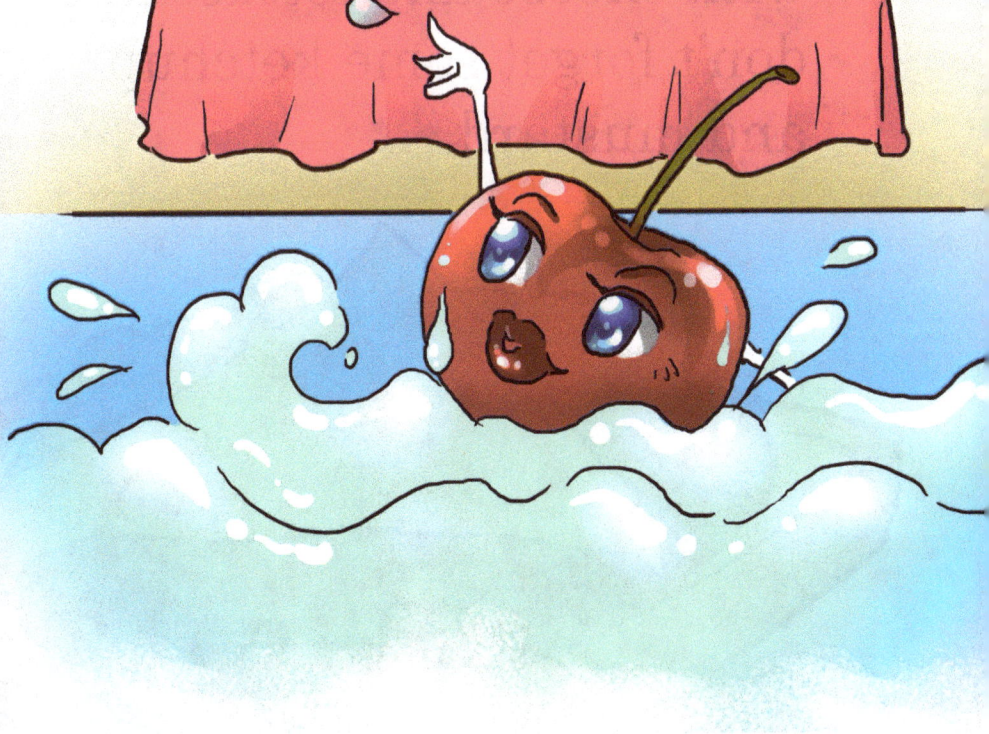

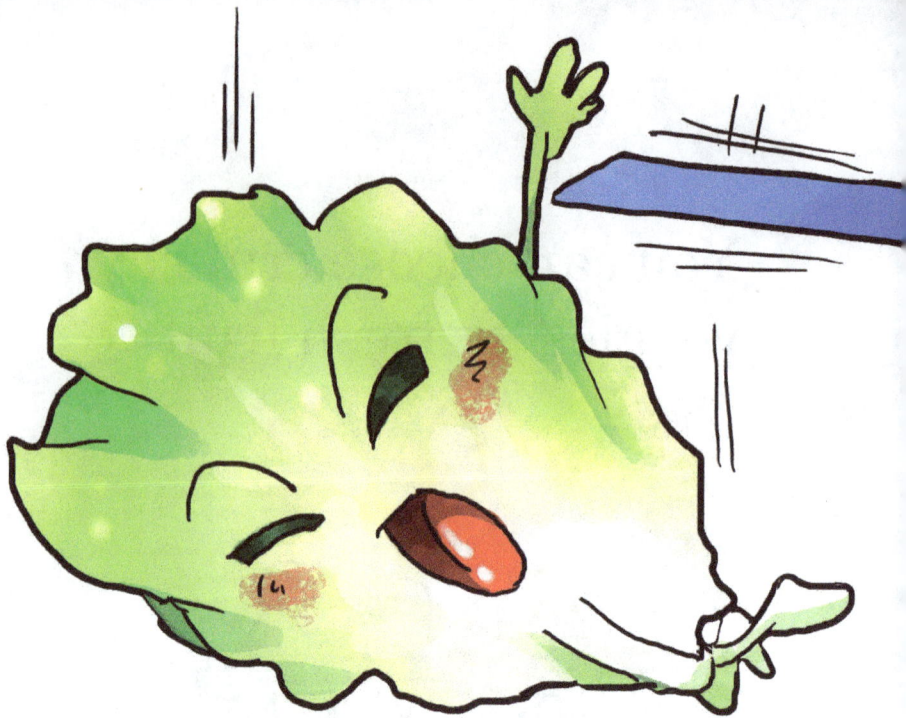

You can choose turkey burger with cheese and lettuce and don't forget some ketchup and mustard.

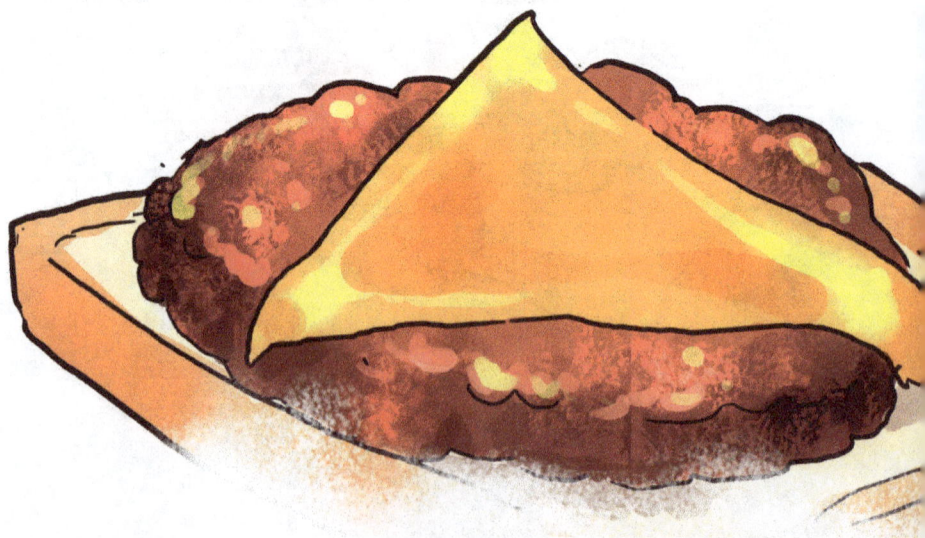

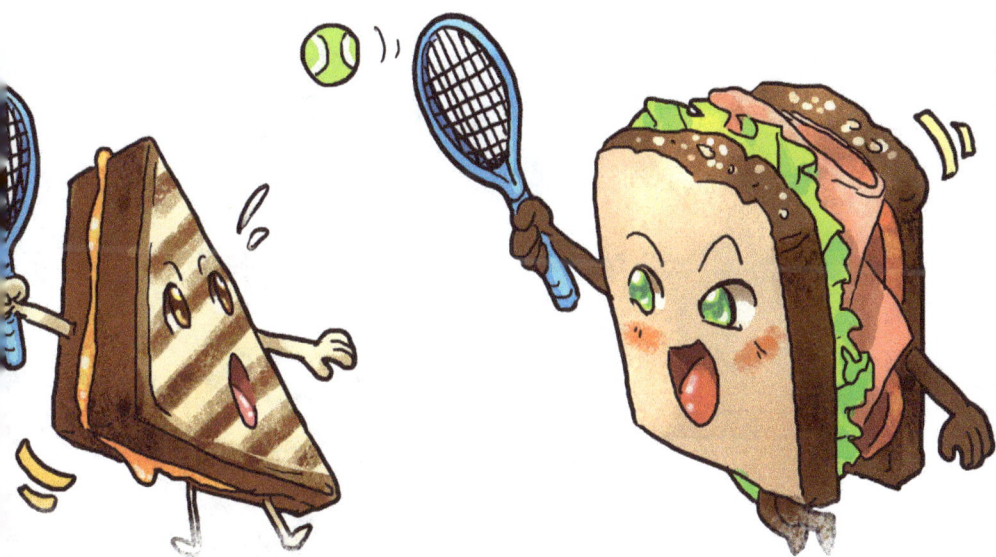

How about a chicken
sandwich with tomato
and mayonnaise?

You can have pizza with
your favorite toppings,

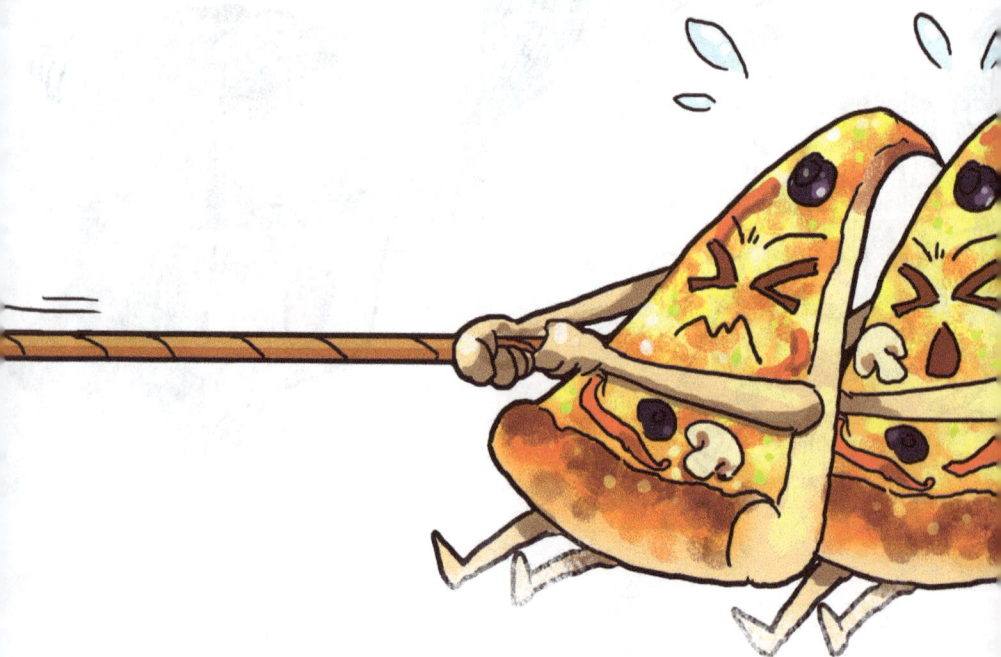

of course, chicken wings
are always near.

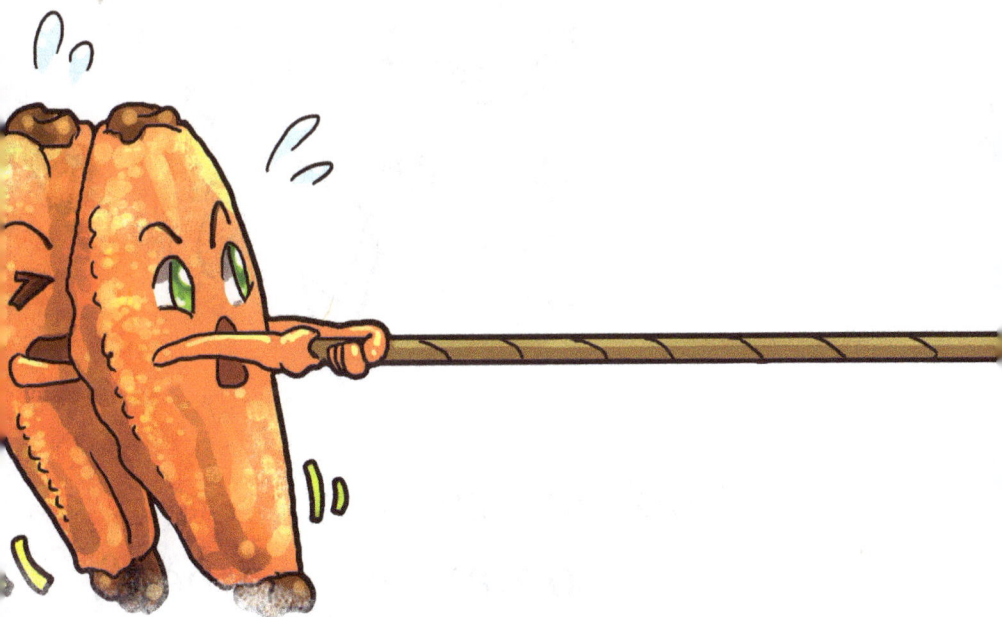

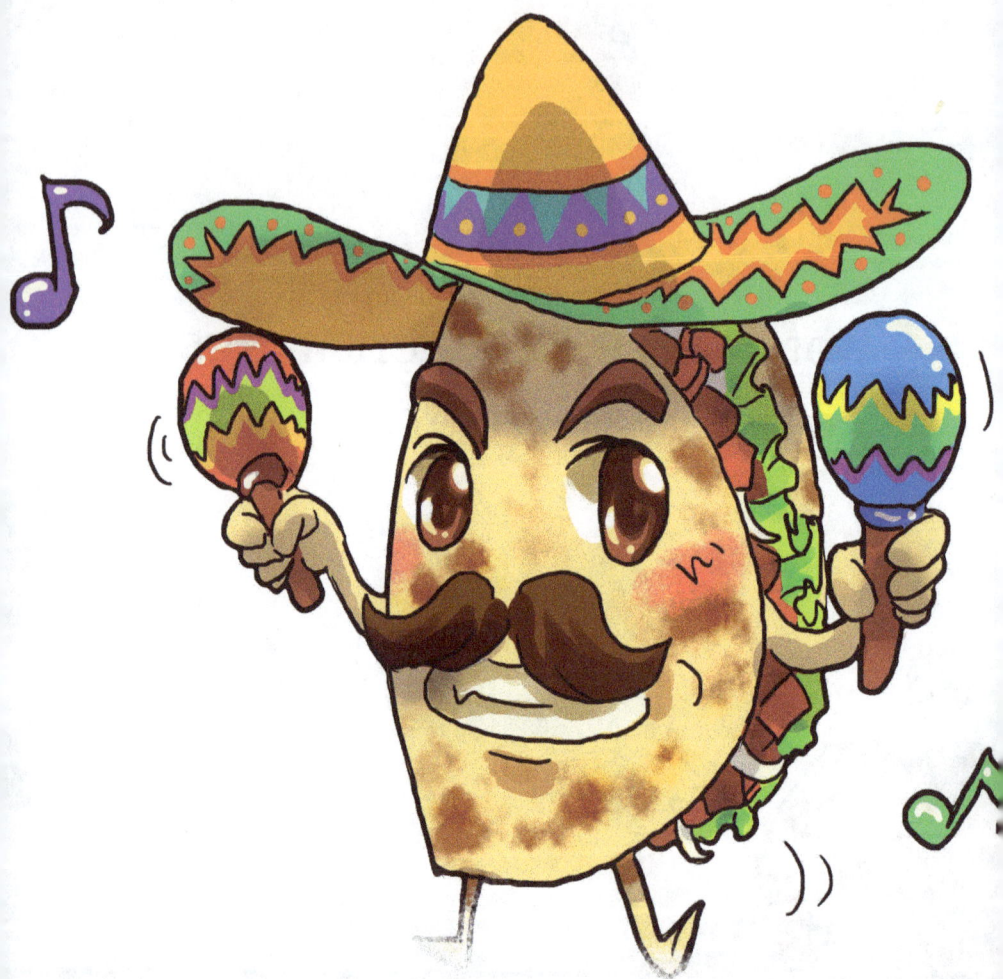

You can try soft taco
with tomatoes and beef.

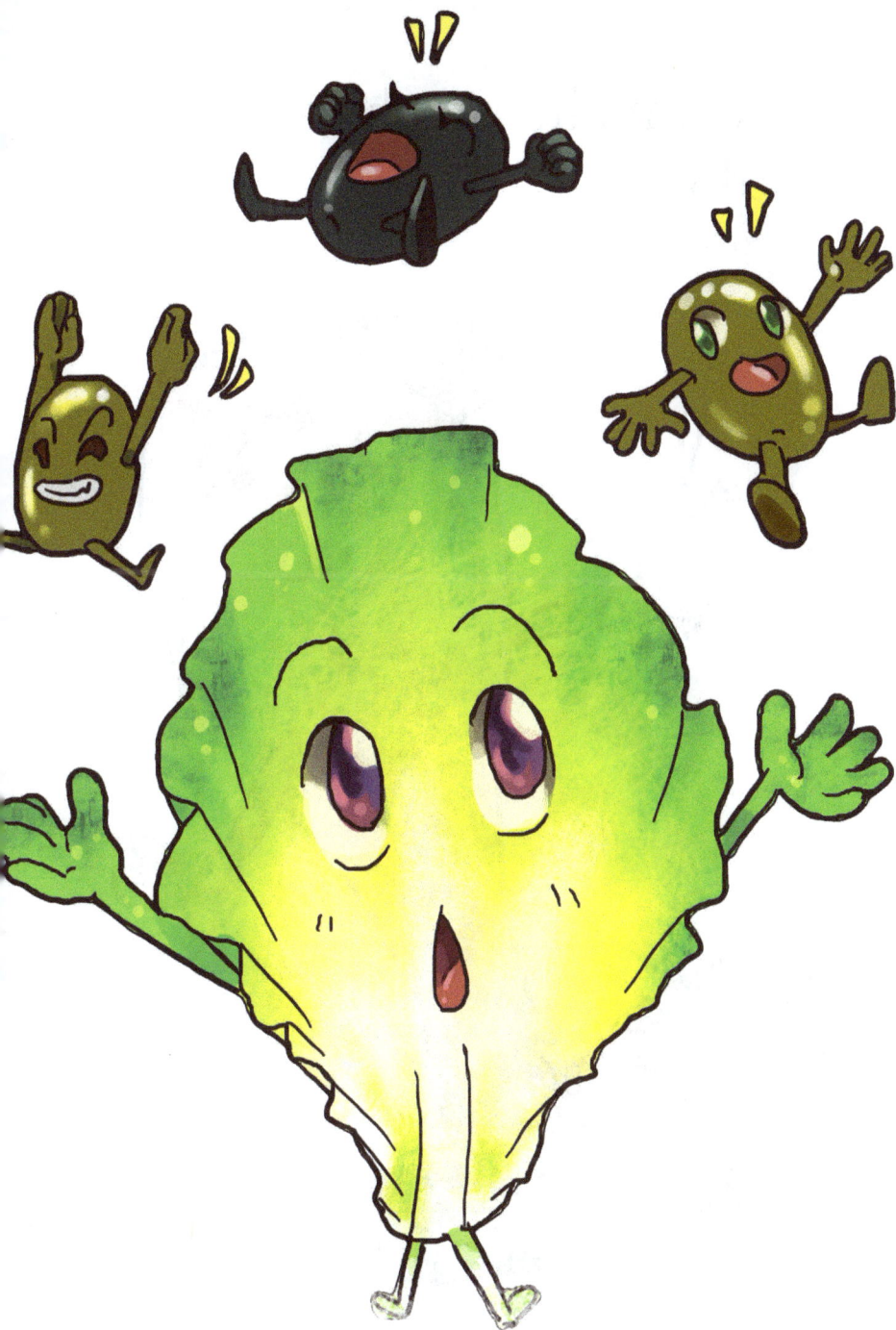

And yes, there is
hard taco with turkey.

You can choose chicken hotdogs.

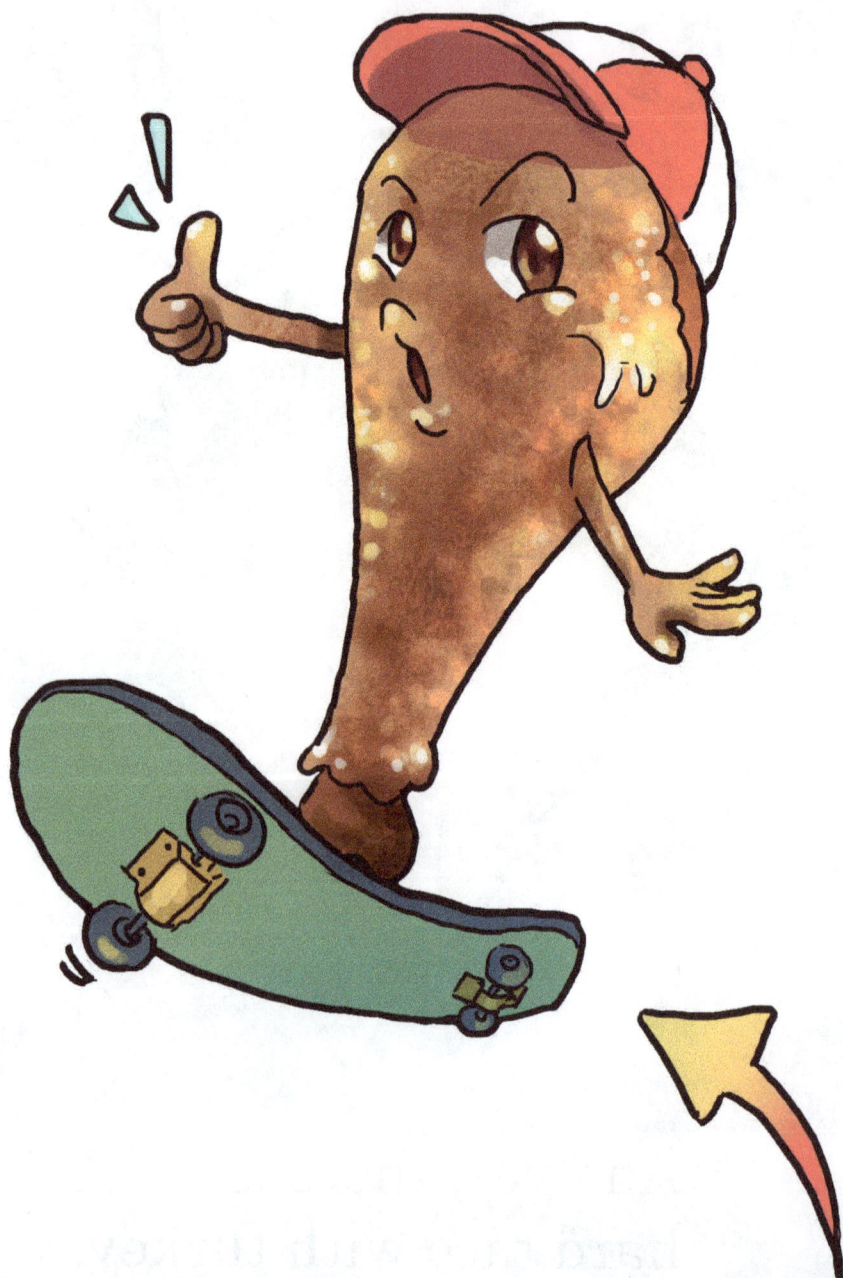

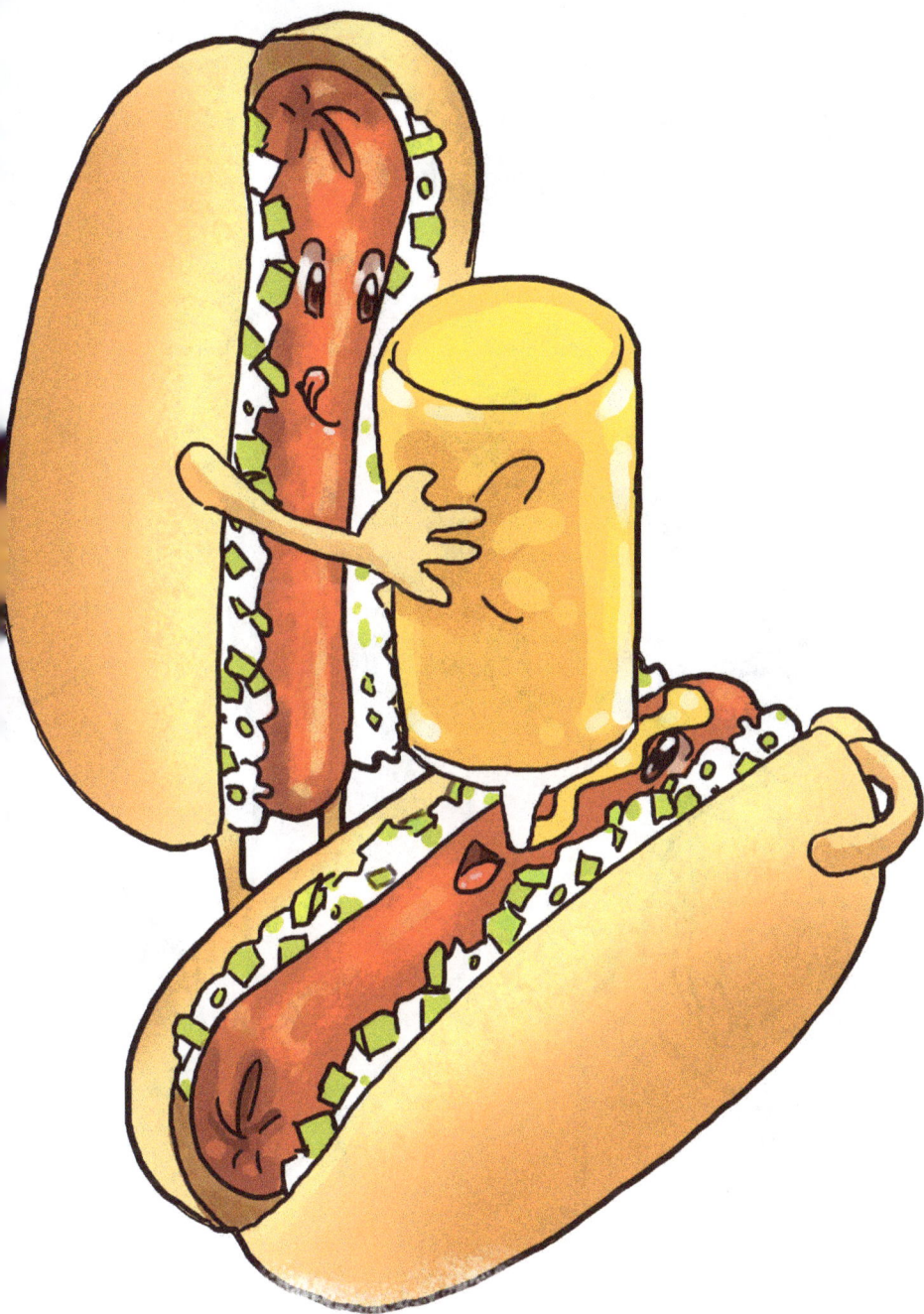

Oh yes, turkey hotdogs
are cool too.

Fish sticks are always
a great treat.

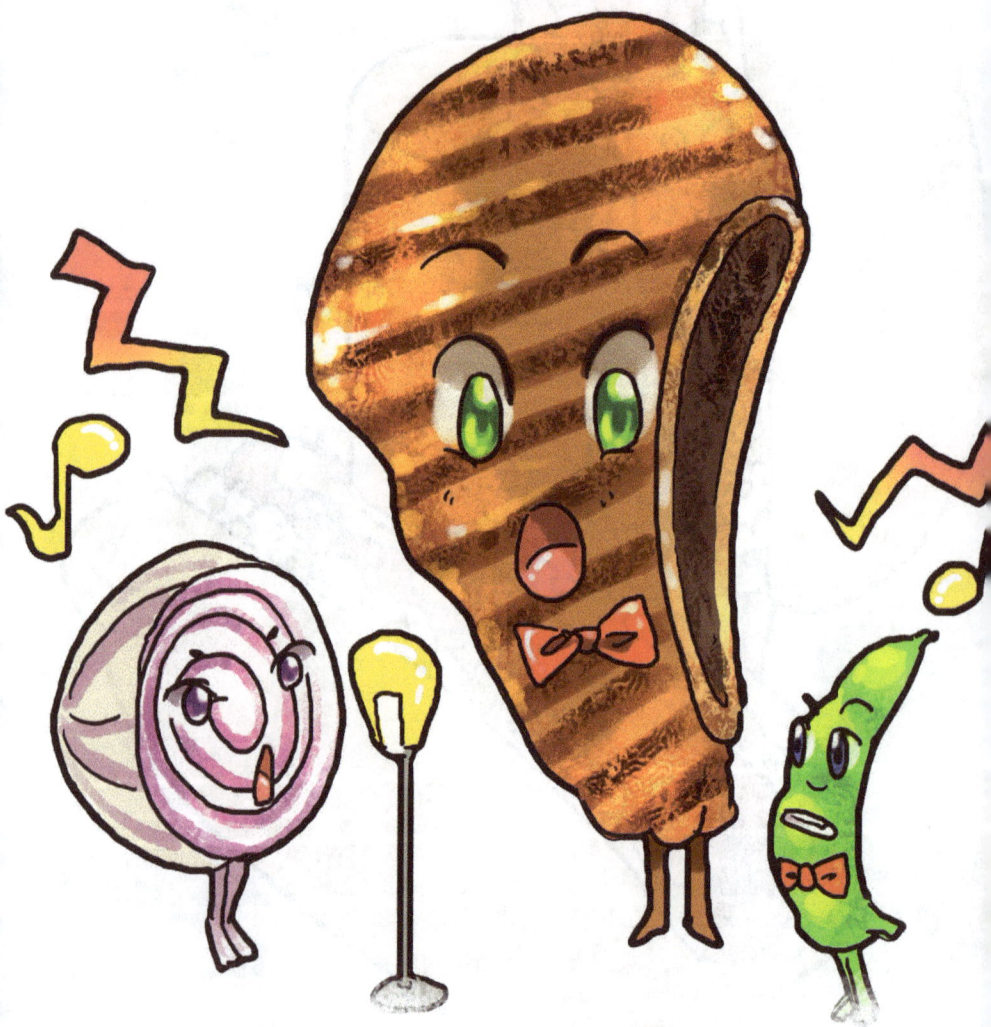

So too is a delicious
salmon patty, so tasty
to eat.

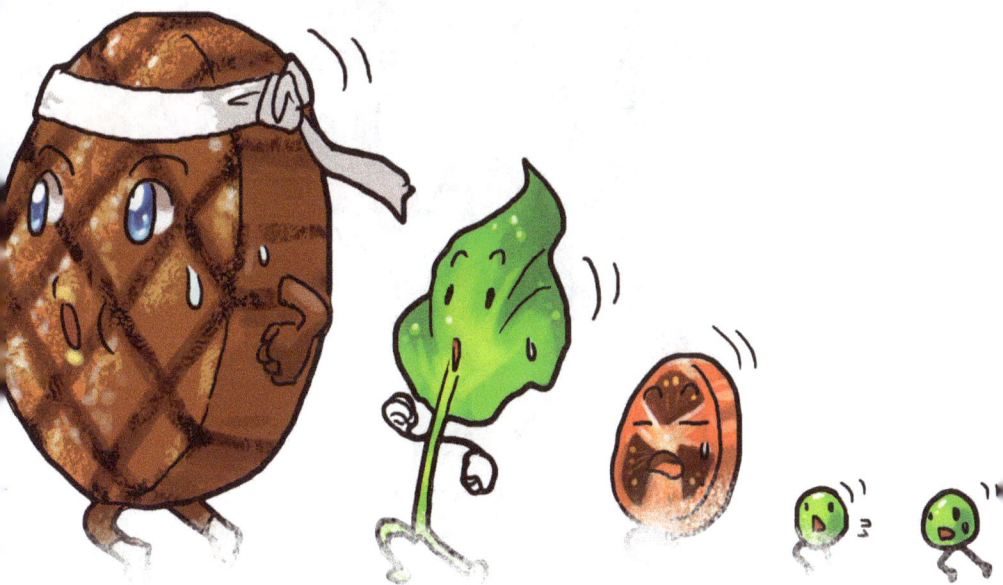

Have you tried sweet potato french fries so crunchy and tasty too?

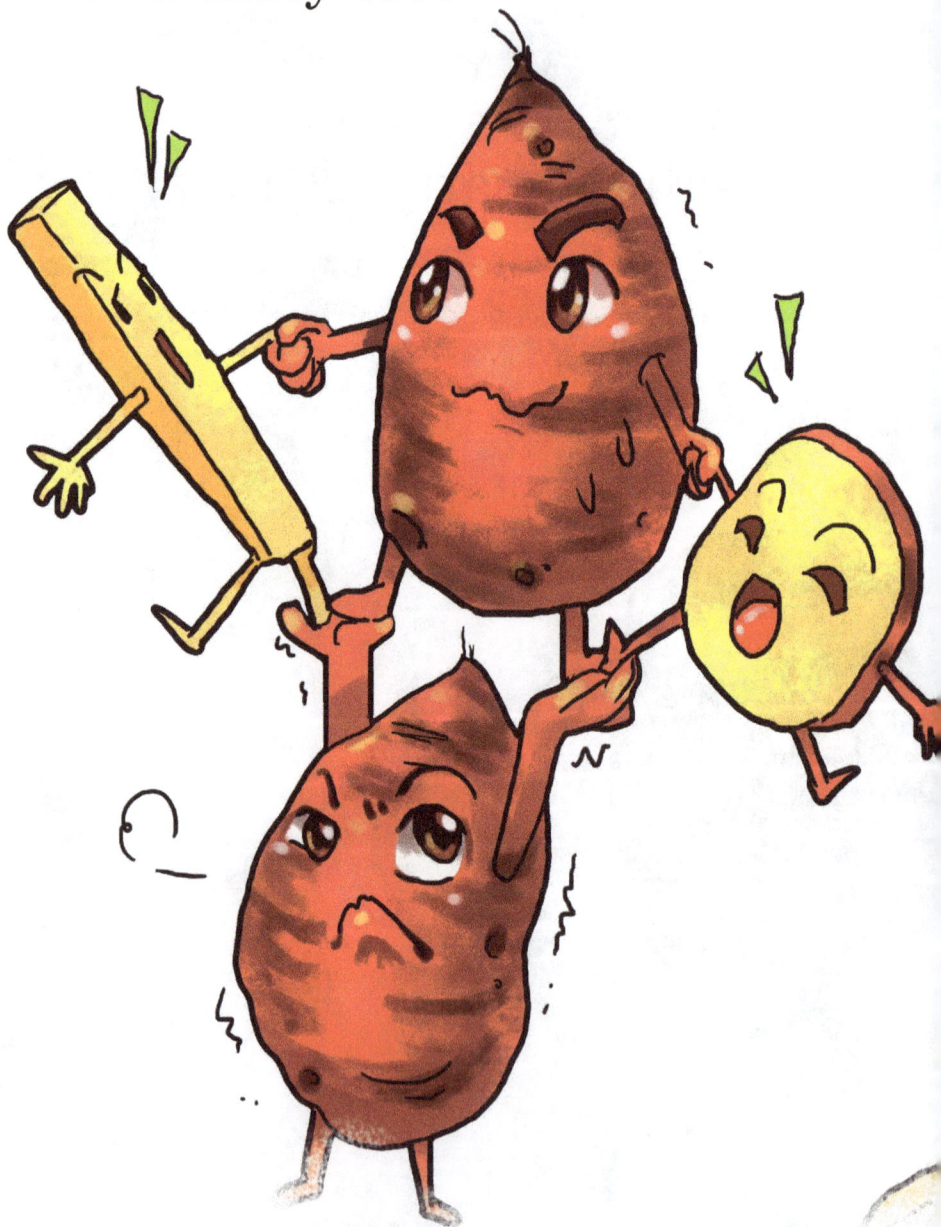

You can choose spinach noodles, or brown rice. They are great with some hot turkey sauce.

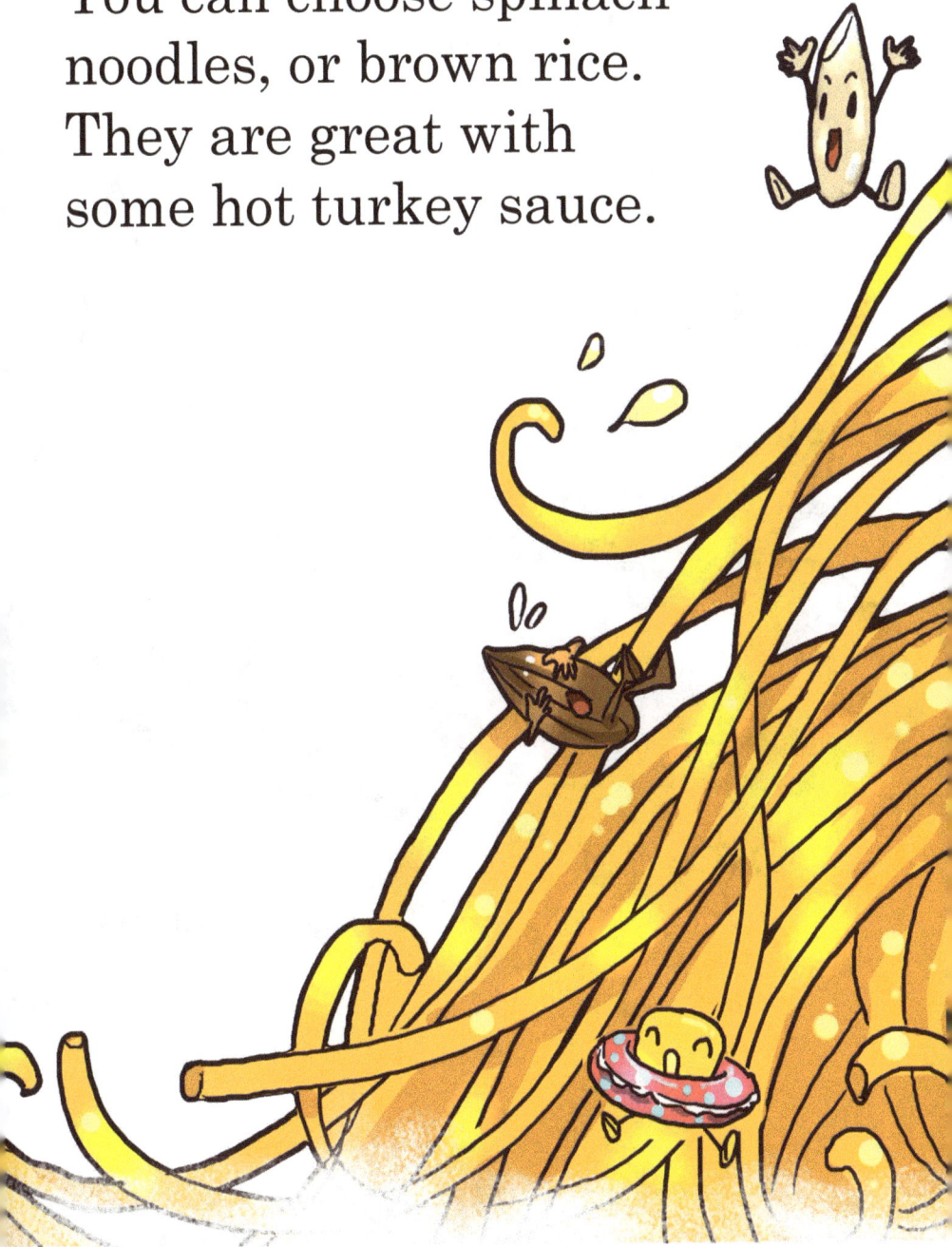

A fresh rice crispy treat
may fill you up.

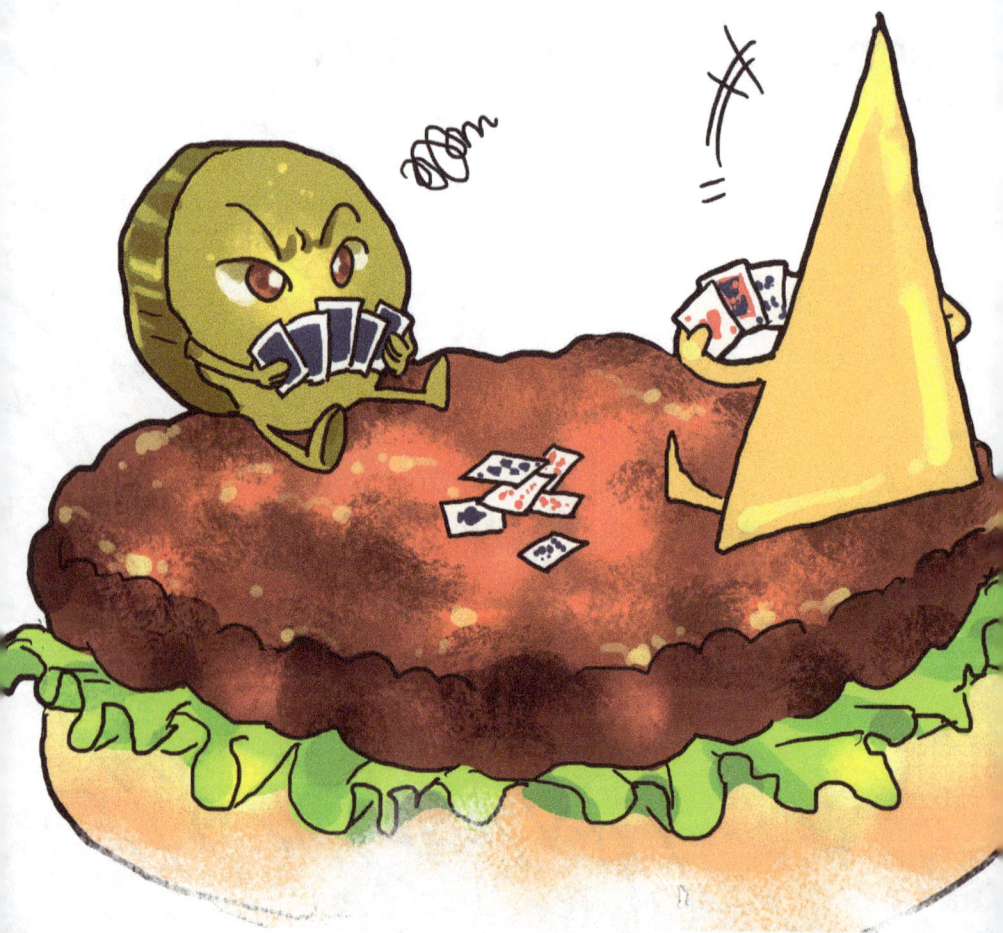

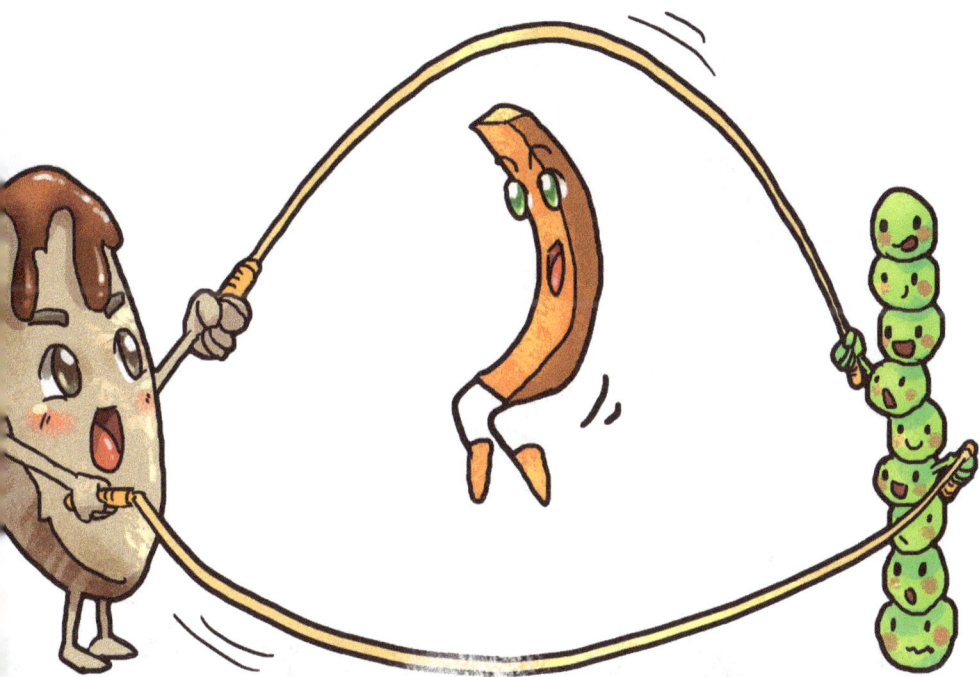

Just don't forget there
are also carrots and peas,

Eating healthy makes
you feel oh so good!

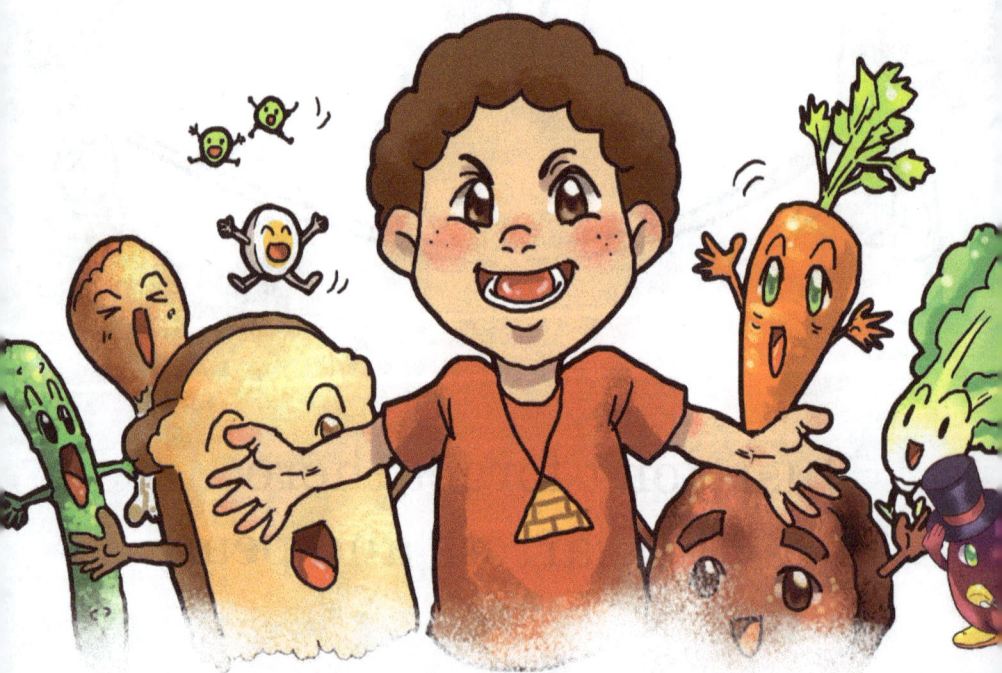

Discussion questions:

What do you think Healthy Ben will choose to eat?

What would you choose?

What are some of your favorite foods or meals?

What's your favorite breakfast food? Why do you like it?

Did you ever have breakfast foods for dinner (like pancakes)? Try it!

What kind of food would you like to try?

What's your favorite way to eat potatoes? Baked? Hash browns? Boiled? French fried? Mashed?

DID YOU KNOW?

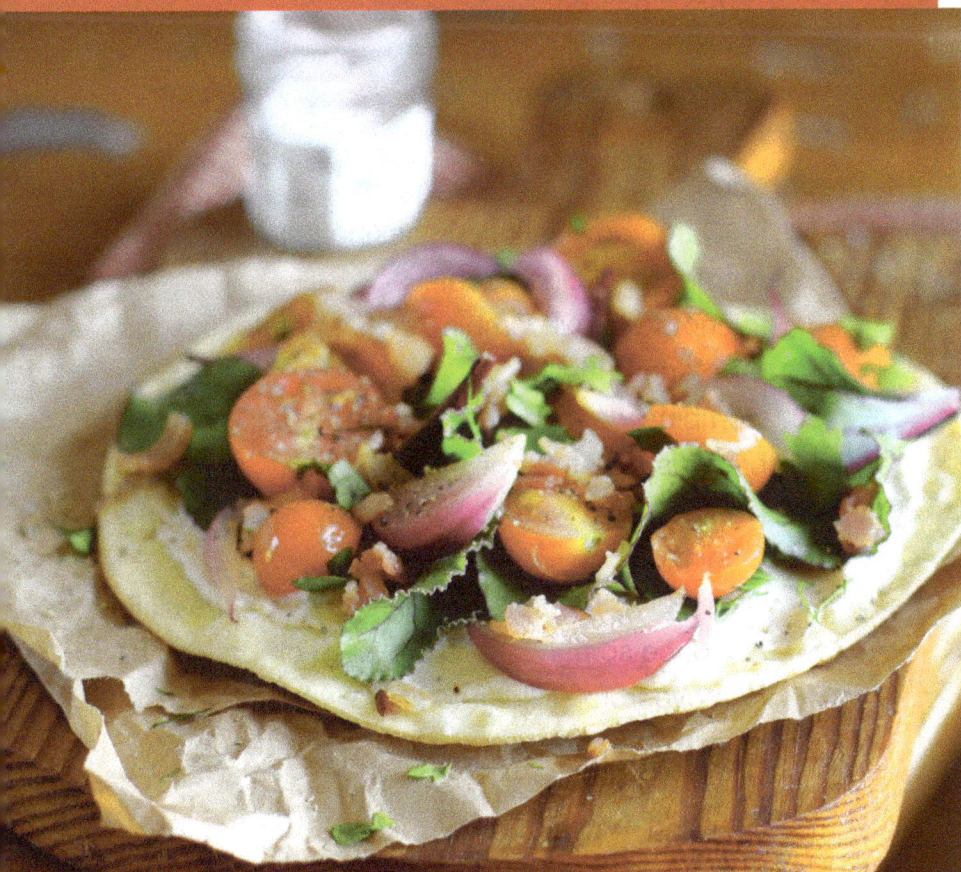

SWEET POTATO PANCAKES

Ingredients:
- 1 ½ cups of all-purpose flour
- 3 ½ teaspoons of baking powder
- 1 teaspoon of salt
- ½ teaspoon of ground nutmeg
- ½ teaspoon of cinnamon
- 1 ¼ cups of cooked sweet potatoes – mashed
- 2 eggs – beaten
- 1 ½ cups of milk
- ¼ cup of butter – melted

Preparation:
1. In a large bowl mix flour, baking powder, salt, nutmeg, and cinnamon.
2. In another bowl combine sweet potatoes, eggs, milk, and butter.
3. Combine wet and dry ingredients, and stir until batter is moist.
4. Grease skillet with cooking spray, and turn on to medium heat.
5. Drop batter by tablespoons and fry on the skillet.
6. Flip once so pancake is browned on both sides.
7. Remove from skillet and serve with maple syrup or cinnamon sugar.

Makes about 24 pancakes.

DID YOU KNOW...?

- Sweet potatoes have lots of fiber, especially with the skin on.

- Sweet potatoes have nutrients like potassium, iron, and vitamin B-6.

- Sweet potatoes are the official vegetable for North Carolina.

- Sweet potatoes can be:
  - ◈ Baked
  - ◈ Steamed
  - ◈ Boiled
  - ◈ Micro-waved
  - ◈ Fried
  - ◈ Juiced
  - ◈ Pureed
  - ◈ Eaten raw

- George Washington grew sweet potatoes on his farm in Virginia.

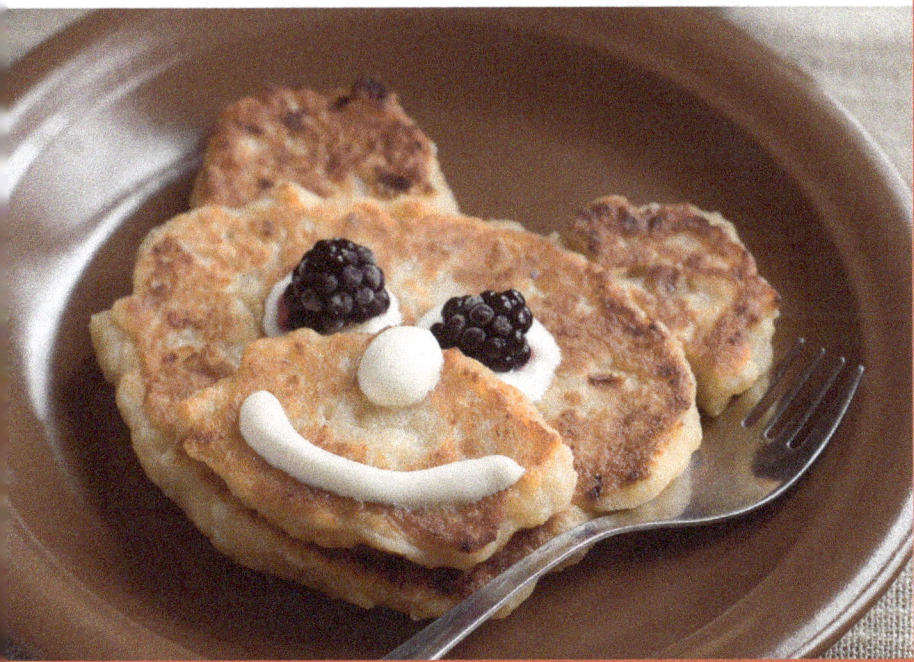

PIGGY BUNS

Ingredients:

- 1 apple – diced
- 2 eggs – beaten
- 1 cup of milk
- ½ tablespoon of cinnamon
- 8 whole wheat hot dog buns
- 1 cup of cornflakes – crushed
- 8 turkey sausage links

Preparation:

1. Prepare sausage according to package directions and set aside.
2. Crush cornflakes on a plate and set aside.
3. Crack egg in bowl, add milk, and cinnamon. Beat well.
4. Grease skillet with cooking spray, and turn burner on to medium heat.
5. Open each hot dog bun. Dip in egg mixture to cover both sides. Then dip in cornflake crumbs to coat.
6. Place on skillet. Flip once until lightly brown on both sides.
7. Remove from skillet and place on plate to cool. Place sausage in the bun, add diced apples, and maple syrup. Enjoy like a hot dog!

Makes 8 Piggy Buns.

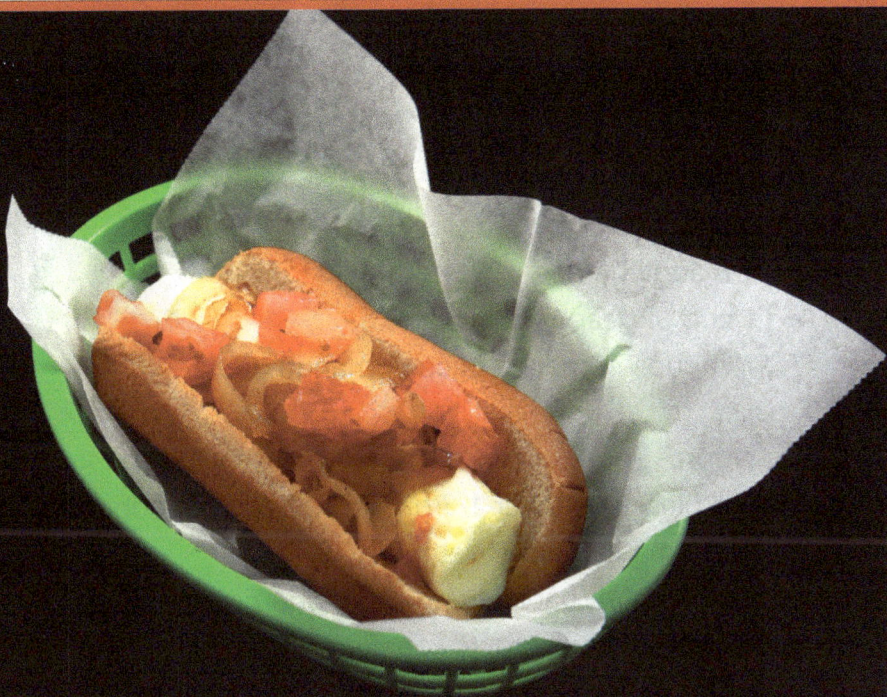

DID YOU KNOW...?

- Don't peel your apple! Most of the fiber and many antioxidants are found in the apple peel.

- The largest apple picked weighed three pounds.

- Red Delicious, Golden Delicious, Granny Smith, Gala and Fuji are the top five apples eaten in the United States.

- Apples are a member of the rose family, along with pears, peaches, plums and cherries.

- One apple has five grams of fiber.

- Apples are fat, sodium, and cholesterol free.

COWBOY BANANA SMOOTHIES

Ingredients:
- 2 bananas
- 6-8 strawberries
- 1 cup of peach yogurt
- 1 ½ cups of mango juice or mango nectar

Preparation:
1. Fill blender pitcher 1/3 of the way with ice cubes.
2. Pour mango juice over ice.
3. Add yogurt, bananas, and strawberries.
4. Cover and blend until liquefied.

Makes about 6 servings.

DID YOU KNOW...?

- Bananas, apples, and watermelons float in water.
- The average American eats 27 pounds of bananas each year!
- An individual banana is called a finger. A bunch of bananas is called a hand.
- Bananas are a good source of vitamin B6, which your brain needs to function properly and make you wise.
- Mangoes are related to cashews and pistachios
- The mango is a symbol of love in India.

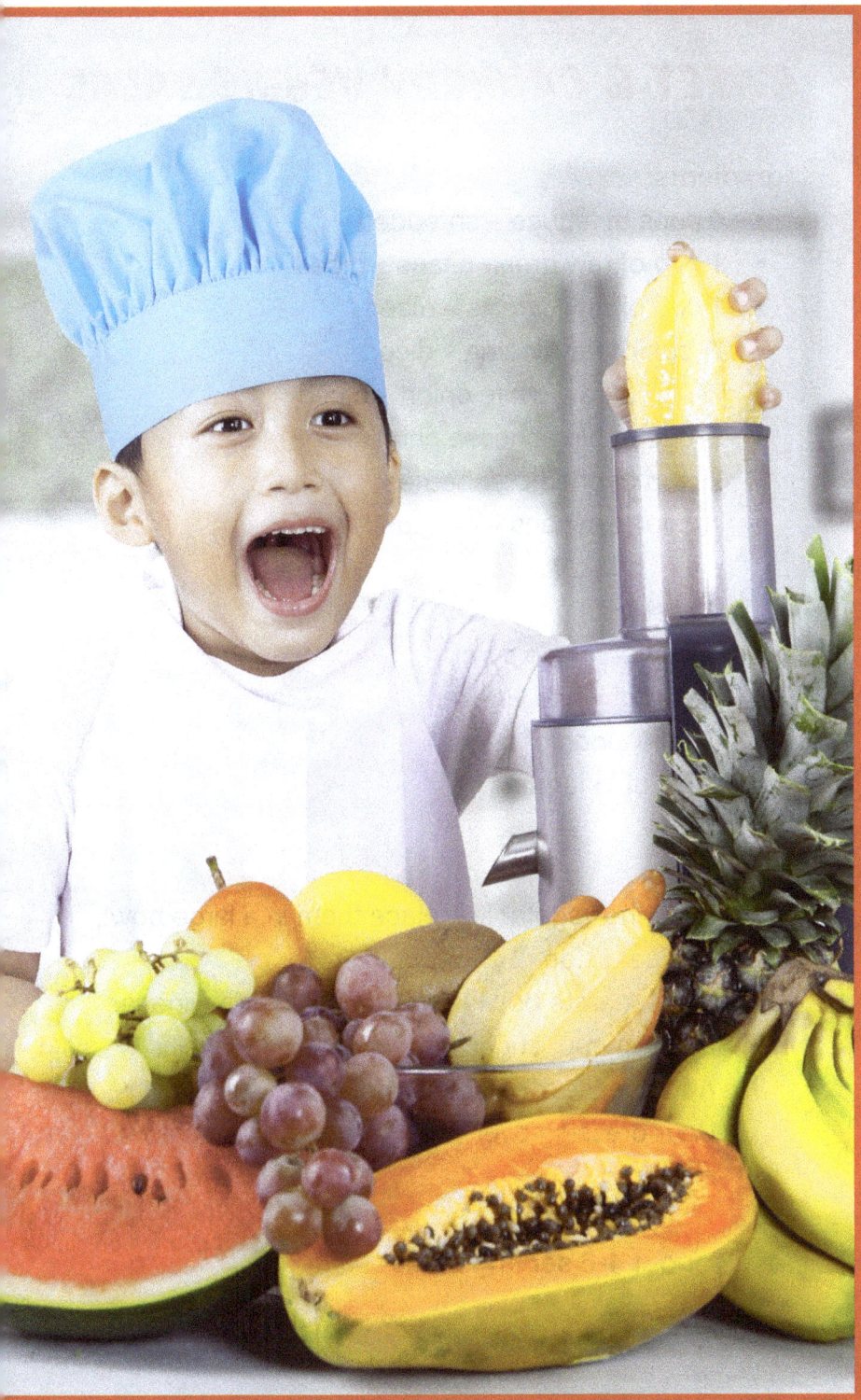

SWEET & CRUNCHY VEGGIE SALAD

Ingredients:
- 4 cups of lettuce – shredded
- 1 cup of raw green beans – diced
- 1 cup of raw carrots – diced
- ½ cup of raw jicama – diced
- ½ cup of raw white onion – diced
- ½ cup of blue cheese chunks
- ½ cup of dried cranberries
- ¼ cup of pecans – chopped

  Dressing:
- ¼ cup of maple syrup
- ½ cup of white vinegar
- 1 tablespoon of sugar
- Juice of ½ lemon

Preparation:
1. Slice the vegetables, place them in a large bowl, and set aside.
2. In a separate bowl, make dressing: Mix vinegar, maple syrup, sugar, and lemon. Blend well.
3. Add cheese, dried fruit, and nuts.
4. Pour dressing over salad mix and toss until well coated.

Makes about 4-6 servings.

DID YOU KNOW...?

- Lettuce is a member of the sunflower family.
- Dark green lettuce leaves are more nutritious than lighter green leaves.
- Green beans are a great source of fiber.
- The heaviest carrot on record was nearly 19 pounds.
- The longest carrot on record was 16 feet 10.5 inches long.
- Jicama is a member of the potato family and can weigh up to 50 pounds.
- Onions can heal blisters.

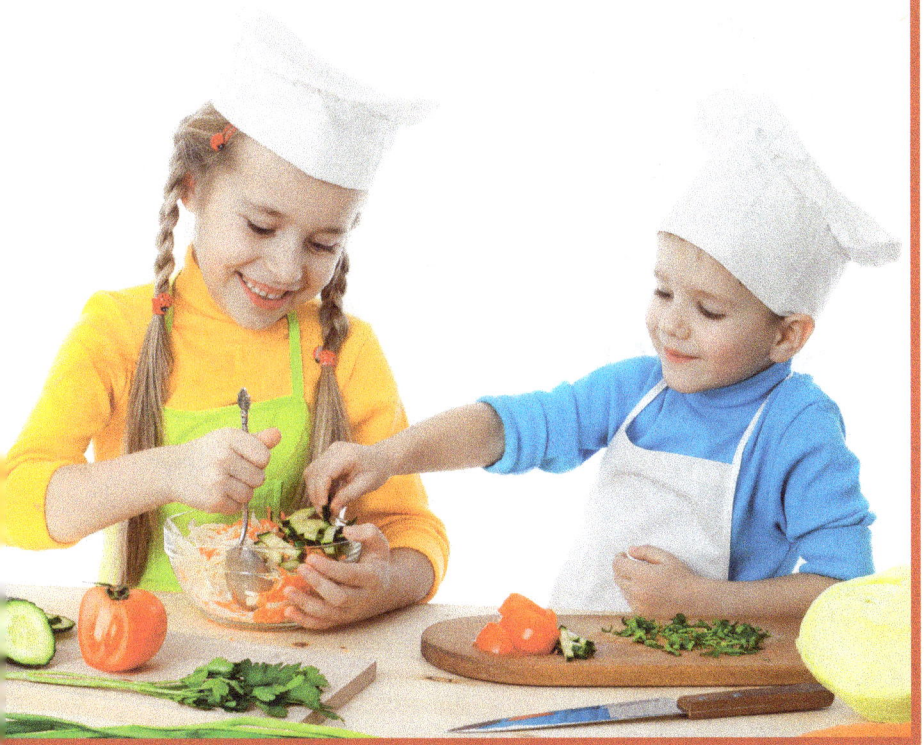

FUN FIESTA SALSA

Ingredients:
- 4 medium sized tomatoes – diced
- ½ green pepper – diced
- ½ red pepper – diced
- ½ yellow pepper – diced
- 1 white onion – diced
- ½ cup of vinegar
- 1 tablespoon of cilantro
- 1 teaspoon of garlic salt
- 1 teaspoon of black pepper
- Juice of ½ lemon or ½ lime
- Tortilla chips – like blue corn chips, or quinoa chips

Preparation:
1. Dice vegetables and place in a large bowl.
2. Pour vinegar over vegetables.
3. Add cilantro, garlic salt, black pepper, and lemon or lime juice.
4. Mix well, chill, and serve with tortilla chips.

Makes about 10-12 servings.

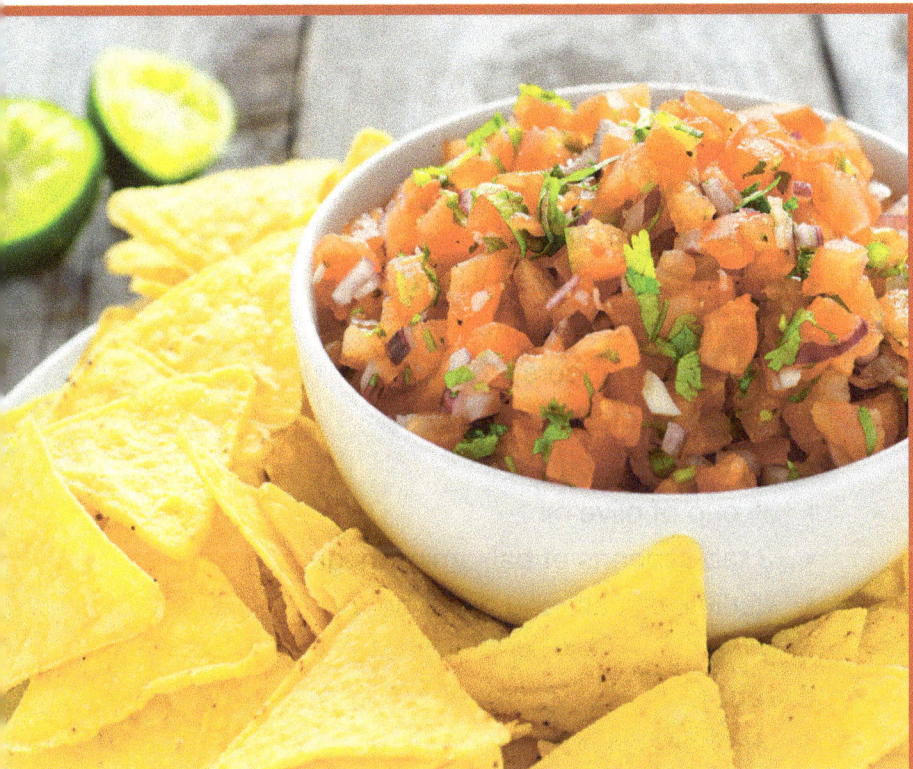

DID YOU KNOW...?

- Peppers are actually fruits that form on the plant after it flowers.

- Peppers can be green, red, yellow, and orange.

- Sometimes peppers can even be white, purple, blue, and brown, depending on when they are harvested.

- Tomatoes are actually a fruit.

- Tomato season is from June to November.

- Onion can help remove warts.

- Onions can soothe an insect bite.

ROASTED VEGGIE SALAD

Ingredients:

- 1 zucchini – cubed
- 6 asparagus stalks – sliced
- 1 cup of baby carrots
- 2 red bell peppers – diced
- 1 sweet potato – cubed
- 3 potatoes – cubed
- ¼ cup of olive oil
- 2 tablespoons of balsamic vinegar
- garlic salt, salt, and black pepper

Preparation:

1. Preheat oven to 475 degrees.
2. In a large bowl, combine all vegetables.
3. In a small bowl, stir together olive oil, vinegar, salt, and pepper.
4. Toss oil mix with vegetables until they are all coated.
5. Spread evenly on a large roasting pan.
6. Sprinkle garlic salt, salt, and black pepper over the vegetables.
7. Roast for 35 to 40 minutes in the oven, stirring every 10 minutes or until vegetables are cooked through and browned.

Makes about 6-8 servings.

DID YOU KNOW...?

- A zucchini has more potassium than a banana.
- The word zucchini comes from "zucca" the Italian word for squash.
- The name, asparagus, comes from the Greek language and means "sprout" or "shoot."
- Asparagus is a member of the Lily family.
- In 1974, a man grew 370 pounds of potatoes on one plant.
- Buds on potatoes are called "eyes."
- The world's largest potato chip measured 23 feet x 14.5 feet.

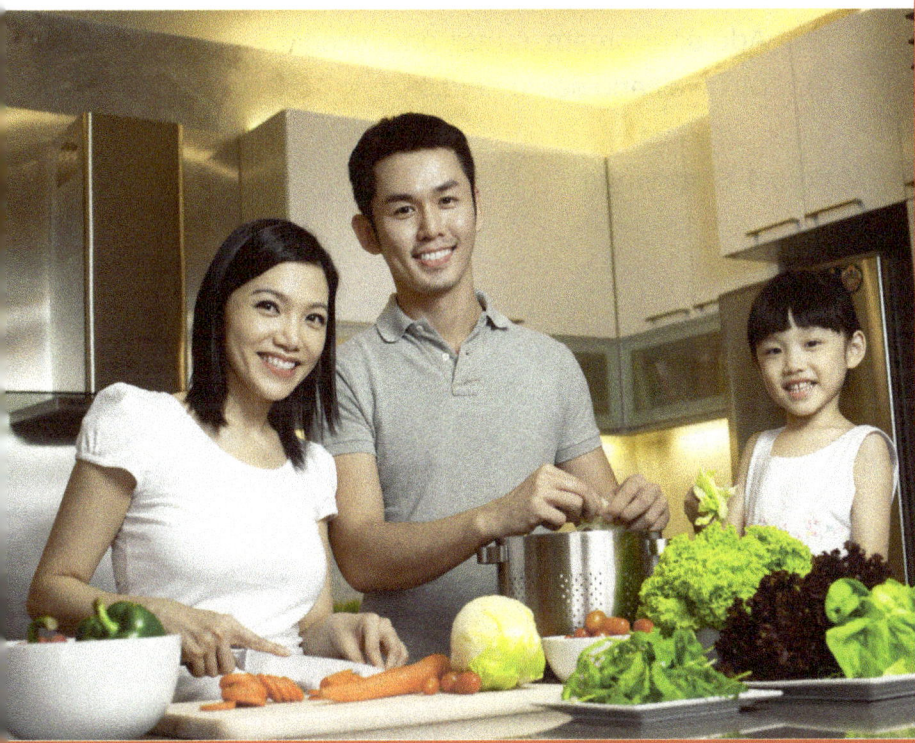

GO GREEN! RAW SLAW

Ingredients:
- 2 cups of broccoli – chopped
- 1 cup of green beans – chopped
- 1 cup snow peas – chopped
- 1 cup cabbage – chopped
- 1 green pepper – chopped
- 2 cups of fat free sour cream
- ½ cup of white sugar
- ¼ cup of vinegar

Preparation:
1. Chop raw vegetables into small pieces and place in a bowl.
2. Add sour cream, sugar, and vinegar.
3. Mix well and serve cold.

Makes 4-6 servings.

DID YOU KNOW...?

- The average person in the United States eats four and one half pounds of broccoli each year.

- Broccoli got its name from the Latin word bracchium, which means strong arm or branch. They look like little trees!

- California and Arizona produced 100% of the national total.

- Cabbage can be purple or green.

- Cabbage can improve digestion.

- The snow pea is also called the "China mangetout."

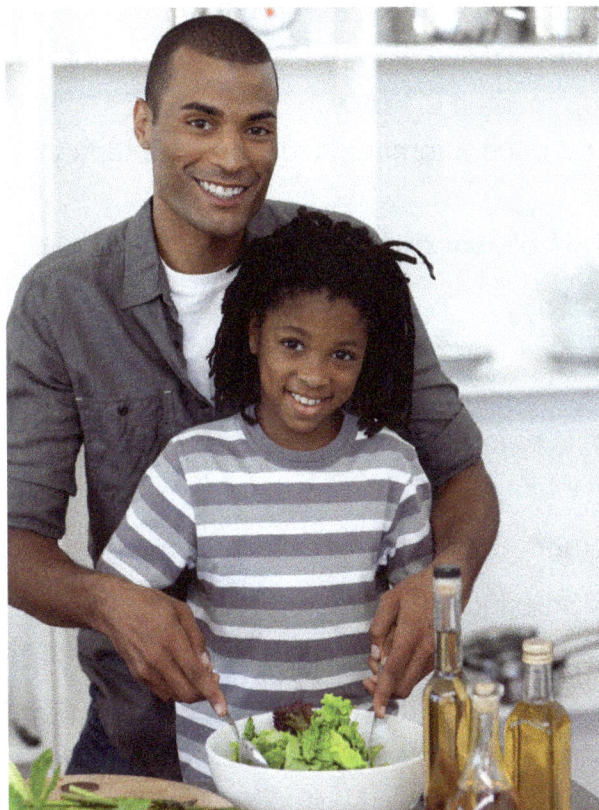

BACON LOVER'S SANDWICH

Ingredients:
- 2 slices of whole wheat bread
- 2 slices of lean turkey lunchmeat
- 2 slices of low sodium bacon
- 2 slices of avocado
- 2 slices of tomato
- 2 slices of cheese – provolone or cheddar (or both!)

Preparation:
1. Cook bacon according to package directions and set aside to cool.
2. Slice avocado and tomato.
3. Toast 2 slices of bread.
4. Top toasted bread with cheese slices.
5. Add bacon, tomato, avocado, and turkey.

Makes 1 whole sandwich.

DID YOU KNOW...?

- Bacon is a good source of protein, niacin, phosphorus and selenium.
- September 3rd is international bacon day.
- Turkey breast lunch meat is a good source of protein. Whole wheat bread has roughly 3 times the fiber of white bread.
- Cheese contains calcium and other vitamins and minerals which are good for your bones and teeth.

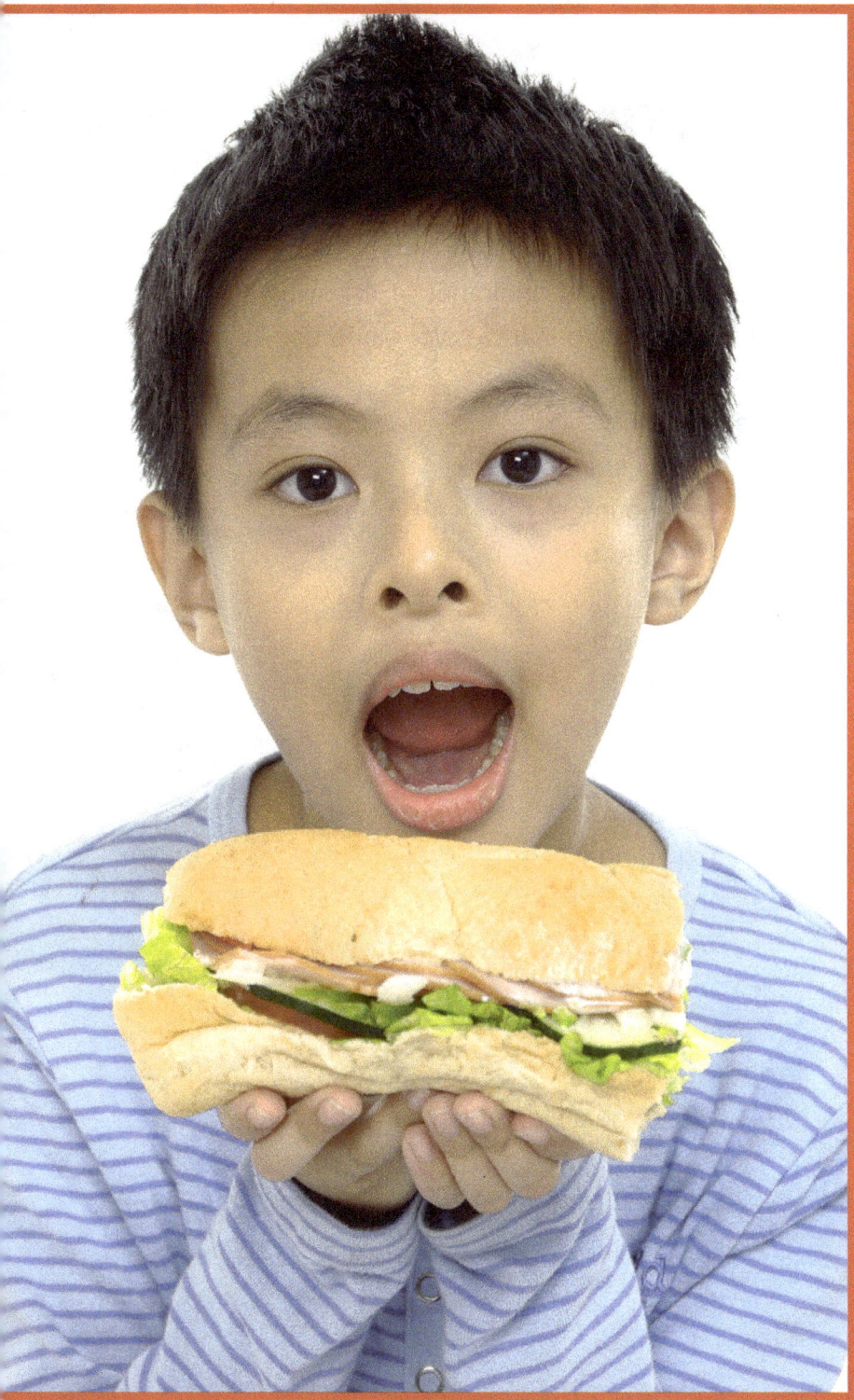

HEALTHY BENJI'S POWER DRINK BY DR. OZ.

Make the breakfast drink that Dr. Oz swears by! This "green drink" is high in fiber, low-calorie and rich in vitamins.

Ingredients

- 2 cups spinach
- 1/2 cucumber
- 1/4 head of celery
- 1/2 bunch parsley
- 1 bunch mint
- 3 carrots
- 2 apples
- 1/4 orange
- 1/4 lime
- 1/4 lemon
- 1/4 pineapple

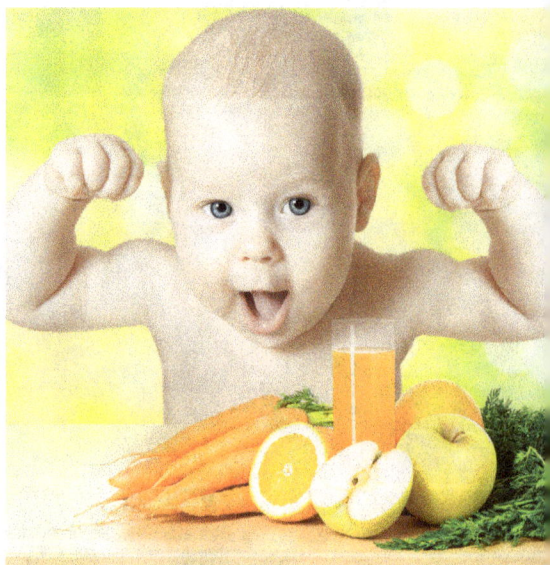

Preparation:

1. Combine all ingredients in a blender.

Makes approximately 28-30 ounces, or 3-4 servings.

DID YOU KNOW...?

- Spinach is ranked as one of the best nutritional vegetables. It is rich in vitamins and minerals, it is also concentrated in health-promoting phytonutrients such as carotenoids (beta-carotene, lutein, and zeaxanthin) and flavonoids to provide you with powerful antioxidant protection.

Celery

- One of the very low calories herbal plants, celery leaves contain only 16 calories per 100 g weight and lots of non-soluble fiber (roughage) which when combined with other weight loss regimens may help to reduce body weight and blood cholesterol levels. It is rich in vitamins (A, C, K) folic acid, anti-oxidant, cancer protective and immune-boosting functions.

- Vitamin A is important for maintaining healthy mucus membranes and skin, and for eye-sight. Consumption of natural foods rich in flavonoids helps the body to protect from lung and oral cavity cancers.

- Vitamin C is essential for optimum metabolism function.

- Vitamin K helps increase bone mass by promoting osteotrophic activity in the bones. It also has established role in Alzheimer's disease patients by limiting neuronal damage in the brain

- Mint is an aromatic herb that originated in Asia and the Mediterranean region. Nutritionally, mint is rich in many vitamins and minerals. It has also been used medicinally to aid digestion and as a healing compound. It is also a good source of several essential minerals, including magnesium, copper, iron, potassium, and calcium.

- Cucumbers contain lignans that helps to reduce the risk of cardiovascular disease as well as several cancer types, including breast, uterine, ovarian, and prostate cancers.